OVERCOMING OBESITY

Uncovering the Roadmap to Your Sweetest Victory

AMOS NUGENT III

Foreword by

CHET P. HEWITT

INFINITY PUBLISHING

ISBN 978-0-7414-8157-3 Paperback
ISBN 978-0-7414-8158-0 Audiobook
ISBN 978-0-7414-8159-7 eBook

Printed in the United States of America

Published February 2013

INFINITY PUBLISHING
1094 New DeHaven Street, Suite 100
West Conshohocken, PA 19428-2713
Toll-free (877) BUY BOOK
Local Phone (610) 941-9999
Fax (610) 941-9959
Info@buybooksontheweb.com
www.buybooksontheweb.com

"America's battle with obesity is not just a fight with food. It is a battle against a society dominated by unhealthy food choices. In this book, Amos Nugent demonstrates how believing in himself, making different choices and overcoming obesity is a journey that can inspire us all to live healthier and fuller lives."

Honorable Kevin McCarty
Sacramento City Councilmember, District 6

~~~

I dedicate this book to my family. To my parents Amos and Sandra Nugent Jr., to my sister Britney Christina-Lee Nugent, to my grandmother Ruth L. Johnson, to and all my aunts, uncles and cousins who truly mean the world to me, thank you for your love, support, and encouragement as I was growing up and while I was working on this project. I would also like to thank my mentors Chet Hewitt, Scott Syphax, and Kevin Bracy for connecting me with the information and the resources that made this opportunity possible. Additionally, I would like to thank my fellow classmates of the Nehemiah Emerging Leaders Program (Class I) for your commitment to assisting me throughout the editing process. Finally, I would like to offer a special thank you to my brother and friend Felix Duncan for working diligently alongside me throughout this entire journey from start to finish. From allowing me to speak during morning assemblies at Gerber Jr./Sr. High School where it all began, to serving on the board of directors for Enlightened Minds Group Inc., and working with me to complete "The Sweetest Victory" program, I appreciate you. There are so many more wonderful people to whom I am thoroughly indebted for the invaluable contributions that they made to helping me bring this book to fruition. Thank you from the bottom of my heart. I also dedicate this book to you.

~~~

TABLE OF CONTENTS

FOREWORD

Young people in America today are facing challenges that are both similar to and unlike those faced by their parents and grandparents. The similarities would not surprise anyone – struggling to be popular, struggling to be successful and struggling to be accepted by their peers, but the similarities likely stop there. One of the most powerful differences is the availability of electronic tools to carry out the taunting, bullying and jockeying for social position that dominate our memories of this period in our lives. The well-documented, and too often painful, consequences of the use of these tools to attack the self-esteem, reputation and perception of youth by their peers should not be underestimated. Many of us who work to help children and youth successfully navigate this difficult period understand that strategies to build, support and sustain their resiliency may be more important now than ever before.

In *Overcoming Obesity*, educator and advocate Amos Nugent III uses his real-life experience to develop sage advice for those doing this important work. His story is at times painfully revealing, and it resonates with his sense of the cause and effects of his personal struggles. But don't read too much into the specifics of his journey; the power of what he offers is its applicability to a much broader set of challenges faced by children and youth today. Presented to the reader in a down-home, straightforward and authentic manner, Nugent challenges all those who work on behalf of children and youth to not be satisfied with superficial interventions. He offers us a new, more complex mission and a way to accomplish it: do all we can to use the omnipresent challenges of latency and adolescence to better prepare our children to overcome the many challenges life will eventually put before them. And, do so by digging deeper to uncover and address the root causes of the social, emotional and physical trauma too many children and youth experience as they navigate through these important developmental periods. Both will require adults to think more broadly and to act more boldly on behalf of our children and youth.

Finally, the careful reader will also come to grips with an important nuance offered up in Amos' personal testament: the potential for each of us to make positive change in our lives, regardless of where we are in the course of our lives. This sage advice may well be the link between improving our own future prospects and those of our children, communities and nation.

INTRODUCTION

Experiencing life through the eyes of another can at times be one of our greatest joys. However, it can also be one of our deepest sorrows. It can inspire us to do great things never before imagined, and it can call out of us qualities that we never knew we possessed. The ability to connect and identify with someone else's story is one of the most timeless, yet most ignored, means of effecting change in existence today because too many people do not understand the power of their life story. Too many people are not convinced of their own greatness and how extraordinary they truly are due to what they've overcome. Too many people fail to realize how much of an impact they would have on the world around them if they simply took ownership of their life experiences, then applied intentionality and innovation in sharing their story with others who are struggling with the same problems they have already defeated. Therefore, this book has been written for people who are unsure if they have a story, for people who know they have a story but have been too afraid to share it, and for people who are ready to share their story but are unsure of where to begin or how to share their it most effectively.

Overcoming Obesity chronicles my life story. It presents my battle with childhood obesity and the lessons that I learned along the way. Each chapter gives an account of different points in my life and outlines the steps that I took to *Uncover the Roadmap to My Sweetest Victory*. As you read this book and follow the instructions given in the "Personal Application" found at the end of each chapter, may its contents guide you through the process of uncovering your own Sweetest Victory as well. I encourage you not to rush though this book simply for the sake of completing it.

Instead, I encourage you to read through it several times until you fully grasp the Sweetest Victory concept and have successfully applied it to your own life. As you read each chapter, pay attention to the personal account included therein so that you can understand my process. Then, look for the life lessons that follow, and take note of the circumstances and situations in your own life to which these lessons can also be applied. On this journey, you will be challenged to recall some of the highest of highs and lowest of low moments in your life because each of these moments are vital to you achieving your Sweetest Victory.

At first glance, it may appear that this book was written for people who are struggling with their weight, and yes, this is true. They are one of the audiences for which this book was written. However, the true reader for whom this book was intended is anyone who is currently experiencing the greatest challenge of their life. It doesn't matter what the challenge is, how long you've been dealing with this challenge, or how many times you've tried to overcome this challenge in the past. This book is for you. Parents, teenagers, athletes, professionals, executives, entrepreneurs, overweight and obese, anorexic and bulimic — it doesn't matter who you are, because this book is for you. The ideas and principles shared in this book represent universal truths that can be applied to almost any situation.

Sometimes we forget how great we truly are, and consequently, we allow life to defeat us. Therefore, this book was written with two objectives in mind: first, to remind you of what you've already accomplished in your life thus far, and second, to show you how to reconstruct this roadmap to success in other areas of your life as well. With these principles in hand, not only will you be equipped to successfully overcome any situation that you may encounter, but you will also be able to identify the specific group(s) of people whom you are uniquely qualified to serve and empower. It is my desire that the information you learn from this book inspires you to do just that.

OVERCOMING OBESITY

Uncovering the Roadmap to Your Sweetest Victory

CHAPTER 1

Psychology of Obesity: How Did I Get This Way?

"Charity begins at home, and then it spreads abroad." – Anonymous

It was the first day of tryouts for the Sacramento Raiders Pop Warner football team, and the temperature was about 90 degrees. Both nervousness and excitement were rushing through my veins as we were riding in the car to the campus of Luther Burbank High School where practice was being held. Thoughts of: "Will I be good enough? What is it going to be like? I hope we're not late," coupled with thoughts of: "I'm going to be the best running back on the field. They won't be able to touch me. I can't wait to show everyone what I can do," were all racing through my mind at the exact same time.

This was my life-long dream. The Oakland Raiders were my favorite professional team, so I just had to go play for their Sacramento "expansion team." The day had finally come after months and months of begging and pleading with my parents to sign me up for football, and I was bursting at the seams. I could barely contain myself. We arrived at the campus, and we entered the parking lot. Of course, I was the first one out of the car because my parents were moving way too slow for me. As we approached the practice field, I was overwhelmed by what I saw: scores of boys just like me, some older, some younger, and some my exact age all congregated in their respective groups across the massive practice field. Feeling a little intimidated but still very much excited, I asked my parents which way we were supposed to go. Near each group of boys were signs indicating the ages and weight limits for the people in that group. But, before I could proceed to the group for my weight limit, I first had to register and receive my official clearance to practice. After getting a physical, being weighed in, and my parents paying the associated fees, I was finally cleared to head to the practice field.

Even though it seemed like forever, in total, it only took about 30-45 minutes for me to receive my final green light, and I was raring to go. It was finally time for the fun to begin. So, I rushed over to my designated area, leaving my parents to catch up with me whenever they could. As I was making my way, I noticed one of the coaches beckoning me to come his direction because they had just started the drill, and I needed to hurry up so I could be a part of it. As I arrived at my station, the coach told me that we were doing timed agility runs, and that he needed my numbers. He then told me to get in line and join the drill. That's when everything changed for me.

Instead of feeling joyful, victorious, and a sense of unbridled anticipation as I was awaiting my turn to prove myself and show everyone who I really was, I suddenly became fearful, nervous, and paranoid. I wanted to escape. I hadn't even run the drill yet, but all these emotions had overtaken me because I felt as though I was standing in line to walk the plank and take the dive into my watery grave. I felt this way because as I observed everything that the agility run entailed, saw how the other boys, who were in much better shape than I was, had difficulty completing it, and noticed that this station was just the warm-up area before practice really began, my heart sank lower and lower. I was already feeling defeated, and I hadn't even started yet.

There was one guy ahead of me, and then I was next. By that point I was sweating profusely, and it wasn't from the heat. The next thing I heard was "Nugent, you're up. Begin on my whistle. Ready. Set. Beeeeeeeeep!" then I was off. It did not take me long to realize that becoming a football superstar was not going to be a reality for me. It hit me almost as soon as I got in line, but it was confirmed as soon as I began the drill. There were four parts: a wind sprint, a scissor run, a back pedal, and a crab run. This drill was set up in the shape of a square, and there was a cone at each corner. Each leg of the drill represented a different run that we had to do, and we completed each run by touching the cone.

The crab run was the last leg of the drill, and when we completed it, this brought us back to the beginning where we had to start all over again. Our task was to complete three consecutive timed runs so that the coach could record our best time. The objective was that with each new attempt, our time would improve because we would be more and more acclimated to what we had to do. However for me, it was the exact opposite. With each new attempt, my times got worse and worse. As a matter of fact, I didn't even complete all three runs. By the third leg of my second run, I was done: huffing and puffing, wheezing, hunched over gasping for air, and clutching my chest for dear life. I literally felt like I was going to die! I had never felt this way before, I did not like it, and I refused to run any more drills. One important detail that I neglected to mention was that I was significantly overweight as a child, and this was my first time being exposed to physical activity of this magnitude. Therefore, this type of conditioning that might have seemed bearable or even normal for some of the other guys was totally impossible for me, or so I thought.

Everyone else was still running the drill just fine, but there I was standing off to the side about to die. I heard the coaches and my parents yelling "Amos, keep going; get back in the drill." But, in between gasps, I was saying "no" and shaking my head profusely because I had enough. As a matter of fact, I had made up mind that I wasn't going to do this football thing anymore because it was too much and it was too hard. Just then I saw the coach approaching, and he was still trying to get me back into the drill. Clearly he doesn't get it, I thought, because he's still trying to tell me to run, and I even think I remember him trying to pick me up and put me back into the drill. At that point, I started acting a fool. I starting crying, yelling, kicking and screaming because I was ready for my parents to get me out of there and take me home. I had totally embarrassed both myself and my parents, and all I wanted was to get away. Within the course of about 10 minutes, I decided that I had enough football and that this sport simply was not for me. I gave up, and to this day that is still a decision I regret. However, I am often able to refer back to this experience in my life and pull so much out of it because, more than anything, this was an invaluable learning experience for me.

As I look back over my life and reflect on the factors that caused me to become overweight as a child, several reasons come to mind. Chief among them is the idea that "Charity begins at home, then it spreads abroad," because home is where my battle with childhood obesity first began. Home was always a safe and loving place for me. However, it was at home and in the presence of my family where I first observed that everyone around me practiced poor eating habits. In fact, I am hard pressed to think of anyone actively involved in my life who regularly made it a priority to instruct me and model for me proper eating habits on a consistent basis. It was obvious that "healthy eating" was an idea that had a relative meaning among my family, and that this topic was always open for discussion. From these humble yet misinformed beginnings, I soon would develop my poor eating habits as well, because neither my food choices nor my portion sizes were regulated with strict enforcement.

For example, vegetables were almost always required for me, especially if I wanted dessert or even if I simply wanted to be excused from the dinner table. However, when I did have vegetables, I either tried to be slick and throw them away, or I tried to pass them onto to someone's else's plate when they weren't looking. I would do my best to avoid eating my vegetables and to always receive as few as possible. The only part of my meal that I usually enjoyed eating was the meat, and then I'd try to finish filling myself up with dessert. Typically, the size and number of servings I would eat for dessert far outweighed the servings of meat and vegetables that I ate because I had very little personal discipline.

To make things worse, I hated physical activity. Running, going outside to play, and pretty much all sports in general were things that I avoided like a plague. I didn't even like to walk fast because my legs would rub together, and I couldn't stand being uncomfortable. I couldn't stand not being able to keep up with the other kids, and I couldn't stand being out of breath and gasping for air whenever I tried. Moreover, I couldn't stand being out in the heat for long periods of time and sweating profusely.

These are the reasons that I always found myself indoors watching TV and eating snacks. Doing this was easy for me. I knew how to do it well, and I was not challenged in any way. As a matter of fact, the more I did this, the easier it became. So, I ate snacks and watched TV simply because I could, and this was especially true during the summer months because I had even more time to eat and be happy. Furthermore, in spite of all the games and activities that were available for children my age, I even resisted getting involved in summer youth programs at the local high school because I would not be able to sit in my air conditioned house and stay cool. I knew that if I joined a summer program, at least part of the day would involve doing something outside in the hot sun, and I was not going for that.

Home was always very positive and affirming for me. My family never made me feel or believe that I was any different from the other kids just because I was larger than them, nor did they make me feel that I was any less significant or important. I was always able to retain at least a small degree of self-confidence and a remnant of my self-worth while I was at home. However, for more than six years of my life, from ages 6-12, each and every day I had to deal with teasing, bullying, fighting, and even social isolation at school all because of my weight. I refer to these years as the "dark ages" of my life.

Every day, I would be dropped off at school around 7 a.m., and I wouldn't be picked up until 5 p.m. or later because of my parents' work schedules. So, in addition to dealing with all of this tormenting behavior during the regular school day, I also had to deal with it during pre-care and after-care hours as well. After suffering through this constant stream of negativity day in and day out, I concluded that there were only three ways to handle this emotional and physical assault that was being launched on me: retaliate and fight fire with fire, tell the teacher or some other authority figure so they could "handle it," or internalize it and develop hardened emotional calluses around these wounds that only time and direct intervention would be able to heal.

To me, internalizing it meant accepting what was said about me, then turning to food as my source of comfort and refuge because food didn't talk back, it didn't hurt me, and it didn't make me feel bad in any way. In fact, eating made me feel oh so good because the foods that I ate were simply delightful, and they soothed me as they went down into my stomach. Eating these foods made me want more and more until my heart was content, and not just my stomach, because it would have taken a lot less food for my stomach to be full. Unfortunately though, there were only certain types of foods that would make my heart content, and they were: cookies, cake, candy, pie, brownies, chips, pizza, hamburgers, fried foods, and soda. This is what I craved when things got bad for me, so that's what I fed myself on a regular basis until I could literally eat no more. There were probably better ways to respond to my situation, but I focused primarily on retaliating, telling and eating. Whenever I would hear "fat boy, fatty, blubber butt, blubbery whale, fat kid," or even a "you so fat…" joke, I would immediately respond in one of these ways.

I must say though, telling the teacher—or snitching, which is what we called it back then—got real old real quick, and it proved to be a waste of my time because I got faster results when I took matters into my own hands. Actually, the only reason I even tried telling the teacher in the first place was because that's what my parents told me to do. In reality, fighting seemed to work best for me even though I really didn't enjoy doing it. The times that I didn't fight, I would either try to keep to myself or hang out with the few people who weren't mean to me. Believe it or not, all of this took place at a small, Christian private school. So, I can only imagine what other overweight and obese youth might have endured at public elementary schools that were much larger.

It's long been said that all people will eventually start believing and acting out whatever they hear or repeat to themselves most often, and I totally agree with this statement. For me, hearing this negativity on a daily basis only caused me to become less and less secure in my physical appearance; I already knew I was fat, but I really started believing that there was nothing I could do about it. Whenever people picked at my "sore spot," this caused me to feel like a social misfit, and it reminded me that I wasn't good enough to benefit from the many "privileges" that came with being skinny, cool, and attractive. In particular, I was affected most profoundly by my inability to approach young ladies whom I thought were attractive because I rarely felt that I was "qualified enough" to talk to girls of this caliber. I always feared being criticized and rejected. Fast forward to high school. Long after I had lost all the weight, these internal wounds yet ran deep, and my self-confidence was still very low. I still could not bring myself to talk to girls because all I could ever see were all the reasons that would make them say no if I were to approach one and ask her out on a date or for her phone number. I was very insecure. However, from the outside, hardly anyone could tell because I talked a good game, and I made it seem like I walked a good game as well. In fact, some people might have even considered me to be both cocky and arrogant because of the way I carried myself.

What I didn't know then but what I do know now is that cockiness and arrogance are nothing more than an advanced, more sophisticated expression of insecurity. When people like me try so hard to make it seem like we have everything together in every area of our life, especially in the areas that carry the most weight among our peers, it's really these people who have it together the least. We are the people who are actually trying our hardest to hide something about ourselves that we don't want anyone else to know about. Sometimes this can be expressed through our ridicule and criticism of others, while other times it is observed in the way that we carry ourselves. Often we are socially and emotionally underdeveloped even though our age and our physical appearance portray us as being much more mature and well-adjusted. In reality, our coping skills and our self-image are still at an infantile or early childhood level, and we are still trying to discover who we are and who we want to be. In addition, when you factor in jealousy as the fuel that further ignites the fire of insecurity, I speak from first-hand experience when I say that seeing someone else with the very person or thing(s) that you wanted or felt that you rightfully deserved is the worst feeling ever. It's like the straw that finally breaks the camel's back or the final nail that seals the coffin because not only has your fear and insecurity paralyzed you from taking action, but you are now mad at someone else because they did act and you are now left without.

When it comes to jealousy and insecurity, age is irrelevant. These two emotions can wreak havoc on anyone, and it usually affects people in very similar ways. People who have been overtaken with jealousy and insecurity haven't taken the time, or perhaps they haven't learned how, to go back and confront the initial situations and circumstances in their lives that caused them to first become insecure and self-conscious. We haven't realized that we must detach our identity and our self-worth from the goal that's always just out of our reach or that we always fall short of achieving in order to properly deal with our fear of rejection. We haven't empowered ourselves to believe that we're good enough or worthy enough to achieve our goal and fulfill our ultimate desire.

These were the emotions that held me back for the longest time. However, my goal of getting girls eventually became so important to me that it gave me clarity of vision and enabled me to identify what my greatest barrier was: my weight. Additionally, my desire to achieve my goal became so strong that it inspired me to develop a plan for overcoming this barrier (get skinny at all costs) and to focus all my time and energy on executing that plan. My plan consisted of tackling the seeds of doubt, fear, and inadequacy that had taken root in my mind because it was these ideas that were ultimately preventing me from achieving my goal, and my plan was successful.

I define "desire" as something that you want and something that you're able to manufacture on your own with limited intervention from other people. In contrast, I define a "goal" as something that you want, but it requires full and direct cooperation from others in order to come to pass. I made this distinction because I was able to achieve my desire of becoming skinny within my desired time frame. However, I never fully achieved my goal of getting girls because I consistently lacked the courage to ask the question. It's been said that both confidence and fear are cultivated in our subconscious mind, and that it's our subconscious mind that creates the lens through which we view ourselves in relationship to the world around us. This was clearly the case with me as it pertains to my fears. I did not have enough confidence to uproot the seeds of doubt, fear, and inadequacy that had been planted in my subconscious mind so many years before. Furthermore, I didn't even realize that they were present in my life, nor did I understand the extent to which they affected me until I was an adult.

Personal Application:

Before you proceed to Chapter 2, I invite you to reflect on the words that were shared in this chapter and recall the parts that were most relevant to you. Consider the opening question: "Psychology of Obesity: How Did I Get This Way?" and consider the greatest challenge that you've overcome in your life as well. Now, replace the word "obesity" with whatever your challenge was. If you're having difficulty with this, it may be a little easier to think about the time in your life when you felt *most* successful as a possible alternative. It is essential that you clearly identify the greatest challenge that you've overcome at the onset of this journey because it will be much easier for you to follow along with and relate to the rest of the book, and the content will be more meaningful for you as well.

After identifying the challenge that you want to learn more about, take a few more minutes to answer these two questions: "How was this challenge brought into my life?" and "Why did I battle with this challenge for so long?" Use this as an opportunity to provide as much background information as possible about your greatest challenge, and ensure that you elaborate fully on both the coping strategies and the attempts to improve your situation that you tried early on. Take some time and do this now. Write this down in a notebook, a journal, or even on your computer – anything that will be easy for you to refer back to often and add additional notes as you advance through the book.

Each of the Personal Applications that follow progressively build on the ones that came before it because the information they will draw from you is intended to make this book and this journey real for you. That's why these guided self-reflection activities are so important. They are the key to successfully *Uncovering the Roadmap to Your Sweetest Victory.* So, as you continue reading my story, I want you to focus on locating your own voice and reconnecting with your own story as your primary objectives.

CHAPTER 2

Mind Over Matter: What Is Your Greatest Challenge?

In my battle with childhood obesity, I had to overcome several challenges. Specifically, I had to overcome many behavioral and psychological deficiencies that reinforced my lifestyle including: a lack of self-control, a lack of self-confidence, and no understanding of delayed gratification. Chief among these deficiencies though was a lack of willpower. I did not possess the self-determination and focus required to make anything in my life happen that I really wanted to happen simply because I made up my mind to do it and told myself definitively that this was going to happen. I lacked this absolute resolve that enables people to move mountains and transform impossible situations into their desired reality. This was my greatest challenge. As a child, I was too engrossed in choosing between the easy road and the easier road. For me, everything had to be as convenient and as comfortable as possible, and it was essential that I have as much as I wanted. Most importantly though, everything had to feel good. When you apply these characteristics to my eating habits and my outlook on life, it's easy to see why I was an obese child. When it came to food, I did not understand self-discipline or moderation. As long as there was food around, especially good food, I had been conditioned to believe that if I didn't eat all of it, or at least eat my fair share until I could eat no more, somebody else would get it. I always had to get mine because once the food was gone, there was no guarantee that there would be more anytime soon; whoever didn't eat would simply be left without and hungry. I never wanted to go hungry, so I always made sure that

I ate enough, plus a little bit extra, to ensure that I would remain content until my next meal. This is how I operated all the time.

In high school, my varsity football coach told us that football was 90% mental and 10% physical in order to help the team understand the importance of always thinking *then* responding whenever we were on the field. In particular, he really emphasized this point whenever we made simple mistakes that showed we were thinking with our helmets instead of our heads. He so impressed this point upon our team that even to this day, I have never forgotten it. In fact, I have taken his statement and adapted it to many areas in my life since then because I believed it provided a relevant explanation for the situation at hand.

So, when it comes to identifying and explaining my greatest challenge during the years that I battled childhood obesity, the first thought that comes to mind is my coach's old adage, but with an interesting twist: Childhood obesity is 90% mental and 10% physical. This means that the reasons causing and perpetuating my obesity resulted primarily from subconscious deficiencies in my beliefs and in my thought process that consequently gave me a misguided philosophy on life. Therefore, my decisions that followed, with respect to poor eating habits, lack of physical activity and the like, represent only a small portion of why I became obese in the first place. If the lens through which a person views life is not aligned with reality, or if that person has not been able to make the connection between what's true about one area of their life and what's also true about other areas of their life, then the fault is not in that person's actions. Instead, the fault lies in that person's thinking, and this is the principal message: Our thoughts dictate our actions in response to our emotions. Ultimately, I became an obese youth and remained an obese youth for so long because of the thoughts I consistently allowed myself to think and believe. This resulted in the misguided life philosophy that I shared in the beginning of this chapter: "Everything had to be as comfortable and as convenient as possible, and it was essential that I have as much as I wanted. Most importantly though, everything had to feel good."

Out of this experience, it became clear to me that the focus of obesity intervention must be directed towards the obese child's philosophy on life if sustainable results are desired. This means that the intervention should produce both immediate and long-term improvements in all of the following areas for obese youth: diet, eating habits, exercise habits, weight management, peer group selection, selection of recreational activities, and social and emotional development. This is why I developed a new form of obesity intervention known as Motivation Intervention (M.Int.) to address the growing obesity epidemic because it produces all of these results and so much more.

Motivational Intervention is the process of harnessing and unleashing the power of your own life story for the benefit of others who are struggling with something that you've already overcome. It is a non-clinical intervention that represents the artistic and inspirational use of positive words to encourage self-reflection for the purpose of identifying your Sweetest Victory. Once that Victory is identified, you then can transfer this strategy for success into other areas of your life so that you can overcome both your current greatest challenge and smaller challenges as well. Motivational Intervention is the process of providing hope, restoration and empowerment to people who are drowning in the depths of despair. I developed this intervention out of my own experience with childhood obesity and piloted it with a group of overweight and obese middle-school students to test its effectiveness. The initial trial was highly successful, and I will elaborate further on the results of my study in chapter eight.

In reference to his theory of Auto-Suggestion, Napoleon Hill once said that "in order to achieve any desire, it's simply a matter of developing enough self-confidence in order to make your desire [become] a reality." However, before I knew about Hill and his famed philosophy, in my heart of hearts I already knew that if I really wanted something bad enough, nothing would keep me from it. I first made this discovery when I was twelve years old because it was at this point that I began noticing a transformation taking place in my life. Through this transformation, I began to recognize and understand a fundamental truth about life: Life is all about who's in control. Either I control my situations and circumstances and use them to get me where I want to go, or my situations and circumstances control me and they take me wherever I allow them to take me. The choice is always up to me. In order to take control, I must first be aware. Then, I must gather the courage to follow through consistently until I have succeeded. In contrast, it requires nothing but doubt, fear, and inadequacy to let other people and other things control me. So, who's in control of your life?

At age twelve, I suddenly began feeling more empowered to take control of my life even though prior to this point things were totally different for me. I realized that the largest part of taking control was taking control of my thinking and taking control of my beliefs. I began to realize that previously, when I didn't think but simply responded to life out of my emotions, situations controlled me. Similarly, whenever I allowed other people to influence my thinking, or whenever I responded to them out of my emotions, it meant that people controlled me. So, what happened at age of twelve that triggered my enlightenment? Simply put, I finally got tired of other people and other things controlling me, and I got tired of things being the way they were. As a result, I made up my mind about what was most important to me, and I decided to pursue it with EVERYTHING that I had.

It was at this point that I not only activated my faith in the fact that my life could change, but I also activated my belief in the fact that I was going to change my life because faith without belief produces no results. Faith is a mental and spiritual process, while belief is an action word. I define "faith" as acknowledging that things can happen based on what you desire. However, I define "belief" as consistently taking the necessary steps that *will produce* what you desire. Believing is taking personal responsibility for what you desire by responding to the inner conviction that you must help yourself according to the best of your ability and to the best of your knowledge, while having no doubts that your efforts will yield the results you want. Believing is shifting your mind to a state of expectation because you have given yourself fully to the pursuit of what you desire; it is shifting the source of your security from what you have today to what you will have in the future. You do this because you are resolved to accept nothing less for yourself. The act of believing means developing an unshakable assurance in the fact that your desired reality is going to materialize against all odds, all people, and all circumstances that may come against you.

Oftentimes, faith and belief are used synonymously. Yet, in my opinion, they refer to two distinct states of being: One is reactive (faith) while the other is proactive (belief). Faith is one of the most commonly misused words in existence today. As soon as something goes wrong, we automatically develop "faith" that the situation will be resolved favorably for us. Or, when we are in need, we develop "faith" in the fact that our need will be met by someone or something conveniently dropping whatever we need right into our lap without us doing anything different outside of our normal routine. If they're not careful, the term "faith" can easily become an opiate for people with a victim mentality because they feel so powerless towards their situation.

In contrast, people who believe always have a victorious mentality because they do not wait for anything or anyone else to change their situation. They do not allow themselves to become dependent on external forces to attain the things that they desire. People who believe in something are very resourceful, and they are very experienced at getting the job done. They do not stop until they get what they want, and even after they get what they want, they keep working because they find fulfillment in the process and they want to maintain their progress. More than having faith that my life could change, I believed that I could change my life, and that's exactly what I did!

Personal Application:

Now that you've identified the greatest challenge of your past, it's time to remove the first layer and dig a little deeper so we can uncover why accomplishing this feat was so important to you. To do this, we must go back down memory lane. So, again I invite you to internalize the opening question of this chapter: "Mind Over Matter: What Was Your Greatest Challenge?" Reflect over the single greatest barrier(s) that previously prevented you from overcoming your greatest challenge. At what point did you decide to take control of your situation, and what prompted you to do so? What were some of the challenges and temptations that you had to deal with along the way? What was your experience with faith and belief during this process? Take a few minutes, and answer these questions now.

CHAPTER 3

Food Addiction: What's Causing Me To Be This Way? Why Do I Have This Challenge?

In 2003, during its 78th session, the Texas Legislature shared the following observations from the Texas Department of Health in S.B. 474: "The psychological impact of obesity on children is both short-term and long-term. The immediate effects of obesity [include] psychological factors such as lower self-esteem, emotional distress and anxiety. Other psychological disorders such as depression, suicidal thoughts, and unhealthy weight control are also associated with childhood obesity." Then, in a 2005 study released by the Nutrition Journal, the authors found that "obesity is a chronic disorder that has multiple causes. Obesity in children has a significant impact on both [their] physical and psychological health." Time and time again, research shows that "childhood is a critical time for the development of self-esteem. Obesity is [characterized as] one of the most stigmatizing and least socially acceptable conditions in childhood [because studies show that] normal weight children rank obese children as [some of] their least desirable friends. Thus, the psychological issues faced by an overweight child places even more urgency on the prevention of the problem." This information was presented in an article entitled "Childhood Obesity: Emotional Effects and Sedentary Lifestyles" that was published in 2003 in the Journal of American Medicine.

As I reflect on my experience, the dominant factors sustaining my obesity were my needs to be comforted, affirmed, and to engage in behavior that was personally fulfilling. At school, I had to contend with incessant badgering and heckling due to my size. At home, I was constantly bombarded with negative reinforcement that perpetuated my unhealthy lifestyle. Together, these are the circumstances that I had to deal with on a daily basis. Therefore, I believe these social, cultural and even economic factors all played a significant role in explaining why I become overweight initially and why I remained obese for such a long period of time. According to the National Association of Physical Activity and Health (NAPAH), "although media attention is often focused on the weight of young girls, surprisingly it is young boys who [are] at greatest risk for weight-related depression." Overweight and obese youth are confused and are unable to establish their true identity because mainstream society is dictating that they should look one way, but the lessons they receive at home oftentimes model contradictory behavior. Young people are therefore ambivalent. I was ambivalent.

Ultimately, I refer to this state of being as Socio-Cultural Disorientation because I would often find myself torn between trying to comply with the requests of these two competing groups at the same time. With each attempt, it always felt as if I was fighting a losing battle that I was never going to win. Thus, what is a boy to do, or any human being for that matter, other than sink lower and lower into shame and self-destruction by constantly eating my way into a pseudo-sense of comfort as my escape? This is why I submit that childhood obesity is a psychological disorder with physical consequences. Furthermore, even though I was never officially diagnosed, my eating patterns described in this chapter and in the previous chapters as well are consistent those of people who suffer from Binge Eating Disorder (BED) and Body Dysmorphic Disorder (BDD). Simply put, BED is characterized by regular and uncontrollable eating habits as a coping mechanism for stress and other negative emotions, while BDD is characterized by an abnormal preoccupation with your physical appearance based on a perceived defect(s) with your body. Both of these examples are noted psychological disorders, and the most recommended form of treatment for these disorders is behavioral therapy.

My condition was first induced by my home environment, partially because there were many times my family could only afford to buy certain types of foods, and partially because my family needed the same attention and interventions that I needed when it came to their eating habits. However, my condition worsened the more I was exposed to the hostile environment at school and the more I internalized this negativity to the point that my external environment eventually replaced my home environment as the driving force behind my obesity. I let the things that my peers said about me affect me greatly, and I essentially proved one of the most well-known children's rhymes to be false: "Sticks and stones may break my bones, but words *WILL ALSO* hurt me."

I remained obese for so long because I began believing all the negative things that were being said about me, and I coped with this negativity in a way that further reinforced it – eating. This is important to note because it has long been known what causes the escalation from healthy, to overweight, to obese, and the de-escalation from obese, to overweight, and back to healthy again. However, little is known about why so many youth (and adults) remain obese for long periods of time without ever changing their lives. Nevertheless, even with these social, cultural, and economic factors considered, we are barely scratching the surface in understanding why childhood obesity is indeed a psychological disorder.

Personal Application:

As you continue reflecting on the greatest challenge of your past, I want you to now focus your attention on the various behaviors and coping strategies that you were addicted to when this challenge was dominating your life. The opening question for this chapter is "Food Addiction: What's Causing Me To Be This Way? Why Do I Have This Challenge?" Reflect on this statement, but replace the word "food" with whatever you were addicted to. We all have sought to fill certain voids in our life with different things. Some of our choices were healthy and some were not so healthy. Some of our choices were positive and others not so positive. Some of our behaviors were short-lived, but others held us captive for long periods of time because they proved to be at least somewhat effective in meeting our needs.

This level of honesty is critical if we wish to come face to face with the true reason that we remained victim to our circumstances for so long. So, what were you addicted to? What were some of the choices you made and the behaviors you practiced to fill the void(s) in your life that was caused by your greatest challenge? How did these choices and behaviors affect you? Please provide as much detail as possible on the full range of experiences and consequences that you encountered. Write this in down in your journal or in your notebook. Do this now.

CHAPTER 4

Weight Loss: Ultimate Desire or Benchmark?

As a 12-year-old boy going into middle school, I thought that my greatest desire was to become skinny because I desperately wanted girls to like me. High school was on the horizon, and I thought that my greatest desire was something physical. I believed that being skinny would be the answer to my prayers since I was sure that being overweight was the source of all my problems and the only barrier keeping me from having what I wanted. Because of my age and level of maturity, this incomplete understanding appeased me. It was simple, it made perfect sense, and the path to the "promised land" was clear. However, as I reflect on those experiences today in search of a deeper understanding of what I was truly looking for, I see now what I really wanted: I wanted everything that I was told I could never have as an obese child. I wanted everything that I was deprived from receiving. Even though I often used the word "girls" to illustrate the source of my inspiration, I now understand that I was really using the term "girls" as an all-inclusive status symbol of the respect, admiration, acceptance, and true friendship that I wanted from my peers. I wanted all of this, in addition to having flocks of young ladies around me at all times. I was looking for my peers to restore unto me something that had been taken away from me so many years prior, something that I did not have and something I didn't know how to achieve by any other means. I was looking for assurance in the fact that if I assimilated to look like them and if I followed the dictates of popular culture, I would gain admission into the "cool club" and finally be able to enjoy all the rights and privileges thereof. Growing up as an outsider, I wanted to be "in." I wanted my allotment of social equity so I could have influence among my peers since my identity had now been established and my value had now been proven, or so I thought. I was waiting for my voice to finally be heard, for my opinion to finally carry weight, and for the things that I wanted to finally materialize. Even though I thought it was my ultimate desire at the time, losing weight was really just a benchmark for me. It was merely a stepping stone toward me accomplishing my true ultimate desire: having my self-image finally validated by my external environment. How did I expect this to happen though when my current self-image was built on a faulty and unstable foundation? Furthermore, why was I really looking for the approval of and permission from other people to tell me who I was and who I could be?

What I didn't know then, but what I do know now, is that if I do not have a positive and confident self-image, one in which I like myself from the inside out, not just from the outside in, then I cannot expect others to like me either. This was my challenge: I only liked myself from the outside in. After I lost the weight I became shallow and cocky, and these two behaviors served as the faulty foundation on which my social status was built. Therefore, my efforts failed every time because there was no internal anchor grounding my actions. Emotionally and psychologically, I was still trying to overcome being a social misfit just a year or two earlier. I didn't understand that liking myself meant more than just liking how I looked physically.

This is what I should have been focused on instead of putting the cart before the horse and trying to have girls like me based on my looks alone. In fact, I should have been focused on loving myself from the inside out, not just liking myself, and knowing that everything I bring to the table has great value. However, this is a lesson about life that very few people truly understand, regardless of whether they're 12 or 112. I should have been focused on becoming absolutely convinced of my own self-worth first because if I'm not convinced, it's impossible for me to convince anyone or anything else that I'm worth what I say or portray that I am.

Furthermore, realizing that everyone has a story, how could I expect other people to genuinely like me if they too were struggling with simply liking themselves? Chances are these same people, whom I so desperately wanted to like me, were also battling with similar conditions in their own life as well. So, why did I allow their opinion of me to influence my self-worth so much, when in reality we were probably at the exact same place in our lives? They may not have been dealing with the aftermath of childhood obesity and all the lingering effects thereof, but they did have their own story. The distinguishing factor is that they probably had more practice at disguising the effects of their story and getting other people to buy in to their facade. They were savvier than I was.

This is why high school represents such an interesting time in our lives. Many people are conditioned to believe that it doesn't matter if you like or dislike yourself internally because it's more important to make believe that everything is okay externally, and to simply accept the lot where you fall as your permanent social caste. High schools around the world are filled with people who dislike themselves. As a matter of fact, life is filled with people who dislike themselves. However, select groups of people are empowered by the masses to dictate how well-liked everyone else is going to be. Apparently, the masses are better equipped to identify likeable traits in other people rather than in themselves. This phenomenon ultimately allows the likable people to establish the social norms and mores for everyone else to accept and follow, or else.

This was my experience. I was not aware of, let alone secure enough, in my own identity to confidently walk around campus with pride in the *whole* person that I was – both where I came from and where I was going. That is how I came to this conclusion: No matter how hard we try to fake it on the outside, when we genuinely believe on the inside that we are unworthy of having a particular person or having a particular thing, that person or that thing is somehow able to pick up on it and will always respond to us accordingly. A practical understanding of this statement is one of the key determinants of your success in life. This holds true in your relationships, friendships, career aspirations, and the like. When I finally took ownership of this lesson and began applying it to my life at age 12, things immediately began to change for me. My life has never been the same since.

Personal Application:

Can you remember a time in your life when you wanted something so badly that you were absolutely convinced that this was what you *always* wanted, but later on you realized that this wasn't what you really wanted because your true desire was for something else? Has this happened to you on more than one occasion? What happened when you finally figured out what you really wanted, and were you able to obtain it? The ability to clearly and concisely articulate what you want is a priceless skill to master. It's one of the only ways that you can experience true success and live a life that's meaningful because the first step to achieving your goal is knowing what you want.

However, just like me, it's very easy to confuse a benchmark with your ultimate desire. So, with respect to the greatest challenge that you have already overcome, what was your benchmark, and what was your true ultimate desire? Remember, your benchmark is something that you probably had initially mistaken as your ultimate desire. Think about this for a few moments then write it down. This is very important, so please elaborate in full detail. For me, the way that I distinguish between the two is that a benchmark is usually something that's sexy, fun and comfortable to share with others, and the path to achieving it is relatively cut and dry. Additionally, your benchmark usually refers to something external and easily recognized by other people. In contrast, your ultimate desire isn't always sexy, it's sometimes difficult to share with others, and the path to achieving it can seem overwhelming or even intimidating when you think about all that's required of you in order to achieve it. Your ultimate desire is usually emotionally driven, while your benchmark is most often socially driven.

Perhaps your experience with your benchmark and your ultimate desire was similar to mine, or maybe it was a little different. Either way, I can say this with certainty: The sooner that you're able to distinguish between the two and identify the benchmarks and ultimate desires for other areas of your life as well, the closer you will be obtaining the things that will bring you true happiness and satisfaction.

CHAPTER 5

Identifying Your Trigger: When Have I Had Enough? What Will Make Me Want To Change?

Self-awareness: Things in my life will not change until I decide to change them. When I come into the knowledge of where I am in my life, and when I am comfortable with articulating my current state in a way that's honest, non-degrading, and conveys my intimacy with my experience socially, emotionally, culturally, or otherwise, I am close to becoming self-aware. However, actualization cannot fully occur until I have systematically envisioned myself on the other side of my situation and taken ownership of the fact that this is the *only* place where I belong. Vision without ownership of and commitment to that vision is not vision. It's just a fleeting idea.

This is one of the most profound realizations that I've ever made. Numerous authors have written about this moment of enlightenment and elaborated endlessly on how powerful and how transformative it is. Countless speakers have talked about this idea in their lectures, seminars, and live events. However, I have experienced this phenomenon for myself, and I am living it first hand: self-awareness. Perhaps it was the exposure that my uncles and older cousins gave me to their very attractive lady friends early in my life. Perhaps it was the typical taunting and teasing committed by my younger cousins to let me know that I would never get very attractive lady friends like they had. Or, perhaps it was a mixture of both these things, along with other influences as well, that finally "clicked" inside my mind. Whatever it was, I finally began to realize that I too was entitled to have very attractive women in my life just like everyone else.

This realization first became clear to me many years ago when I was in the sixth grade. I began reflecting on the fact that when I was younger, I'd always received a welcome and inviting reception from very attractive older women. Whenever I was around them, we would sit and talk about many different things, and this became a regular occurrence for me. Somehow or another, I would always find myself enjoying quality one-on-one time with these very attractive older women, and that's when I would go in and make my move. My ultimate goal was for her to leave her man and become my girl – even if that man was my uncle, my cousin, or some other guy that I didn't know. Whenever I did this, they would always think I was cute and funny, but above all, they would always think I was just joking or being silly so they would simply laugh off my advances. They didn't know that I was very serious, and that I really believed that the two of us could be an item. I would say things like, "Why don't you leave your man and go out with me?" or "You should take his picture down off your dashboard and put mine up." I would also look for any excuse to have physical contact with them. Because I was a little kid, they didn't think anything of it. They thought that my attempts were nothing more than innocent and playful gestures, so they didn't pay any attention to them.

Life was great. Being with them and enjoying their company as we simply hung out and chatted made me feel so good. It made me feel special, it made me feel important, and it made me feel like I was somebody. They made feel as though I brought real value to their lives simply by entertaining them. I felt like I could be me, she could be her, and we both were happy with each other just the way we were. These ladies spent significant amounts of time with me without shutting me down or telling me to "run along and play," and I couldn't have asked for anything more. Even though I was young, I seriously felt a connection with these women, and I believe this is why I have an affinity for very attractive older women today. These were the types of women that I was exposed to most consistently, and this is the description that comes to mind when I envision what the ideal woman would look like for me today. Let me be clear though. When I say very attractive older women, I do not mean old women; I am simply referring to women who are just a few years older than me. All of this happened in my early childhood between the ages of 5-8, well before I reached the height of my obesity. I was slightly overweight then, but my size was overlooked because I was young and it was assumed that this "baby fat" would eventually go away. Well, eventually never came until six or seven years later. In the meantime though, I grew larger and larger, and my health dramatically worsened.

For whatever reason, I stopped having as much contact with those very attractive older women whose presence I had enjoyed so much. In fact, my contact with all girls in general significantly declined. It was almost as if my presence repelled them and disgusted them, and perhaps it did. I could never find the words to say, nor was I given the opportunity to establish a rapport with my female peers during my elementary school years in the same manner I had been accustomed to with those very attractive older women that I was previously exposed to. I lived this reality day in and day out for several years, and I believe it ultimately caused stagnation and regression in my social development. Now, factor in the Socio-Cultural Disorientation mentioned earlier that resulted from the constant negativity I had to deal with at school and the poor health practices that were modeled for me at home, and the sources of my psychological and emotional frustrations are illuminated even the more. I lived this way for over six years, simply accepting whatever was dealt to me because: "What more can I do?" "How can I change my situation?" "Is this how the rest of my life is going to be?" These thoughts and others just like them clouded my mind all the time, but I didn't know how to express them, nor did I have a safe place where I could begin to try. What was wrong with me? I didn't want to be big. I was still a nice guy with good intentions. However, very few people were willing to look beyond my size, recognize me as a human being, and treat me the same way they did everyone else on the playground.

All I wanted was to return to my glory days, and the most immediate barrier preventing me from doing this was my weight. So, herein lay the problem, and I was determined to fix it. In fact, fixing this problem quickly became my number one priority because high school was on the horizon, and I knew I had to get myself together since it was obvious that girls didn't like fat guys! Therefore, I became obsessed with the idea of losing weight. This was something totally new and different for me, and it was unlike anything I had ever done before. I had to figure everything out for myself through trial and error, and I had to follow my intuition at all times in order to make the best decisions and take the most appropriate actions. Nevertheless, this experience was one of the best times of my entire life, and I wouldn't have traded it for anything. My inexperience was never an excuse for me because the pain of remaining the same had finally become greater than the pain of changing. I was finally ready for action. But at such a young age, my exposure to exercise techniques and familiarity with workout plans was very limited. I only knew the basics of what I occasionally saw on TV and what I periodically witnessed other people doing in person: sit-ups, push-ups, and running or jogging. So, I decided to create my own workout plan based on these three activities. It all began the summer following my sixth grade year, and I remember it as if was yesterday.

To break the monotony of being at home and being bored, I usually spent my summers at my grandmother's house. Her house always represented fun times and fond memories for me because I was able to stay up late, watch as much TV as I wanted, eat as much food as I wanted, and pretty much do whatever I wanted to do. Additionally, the local high school near her house always held summer programs for youth who lived in the area so we would have something positive to do during the day. This summer was different though. Since I now had a specific goal in mind that I was determined to achieve, I didn't have the desire to engage in all the usual activities that I typically spent my summers doing. This summer, my singular objective was to get skinny at all costs and by any means necessary. This was going to happen because I had made up my mind that I was going to do it!

When I first began, I was intently trying to determine the changes I needed to make in my life in order to experience these new results because I knew that I was not going to continue my same old habits. Almost immediately, I recognized that I needed to change both my diet and my eating habits because they were the key drivers that had been causing my poor physical condition. Then I realized that I had to incorporate exercise and physical activity into my life as well. It was as if my level of self-awareness had instantly been heightened, and I could now see exactly what was causing me to be obese. More importantly, I felt empowered to change my circumstances since I now saw clear-cut solutions. I was able to simplify my roadmap to transformation into two steps, and these two steps are the topics of the next two chapters respectively. I had finally come to my senses, and I had finally realized that I deserve better than what I was currently receiving from my surrounding environment. I decided that based on my personal experiences with those very attractive older women during my early childhood, I *was capable* of getting girls—but not just any girls. I decided that I was capable of getting the most attractive girls. The positive reinforcement that I received early in life ended up becoming both my saving grace and my ultimate motivation to change because I had resolved within myself that if I did it once, I could definitely do it again! I knew at that moment that I had it in me to take my life back. I knew at that moment that I had it in me to regain my social status and return it to the place where it used to be – the place where I enjoyed life and life enjoyed me. I decided in that moment that I was going to do everything it took for me to return to my glory days.

This example shows the power of our life experiences, both positive and negative, and how they serve as a continuously unfolding story that we can always reference at any point in our lives. We never know when it will become necessary, or even vital, for us to draw upon a situation or circumstance from our past in order to find the meaning of and establish a clear direction for a present situation. Additionally, once this wisdom has been accessed, it is there not only for our benefit, but it is there for us to share with others as well. This is especially true when we encounter people who are in the same place where we once were. In times like these, we can use our intimacy with our experience, both the painful and the pleasurable aspects, to help others overcome what we have already overcame. When we allow ourselves to remain in uncomfortable situations, this is an indicator that we lack courage and that we lack our own identity because we are allowing someone or something else to define us: who we are now and who we are going to be, indefinitely. This person or thing has the power to have its way with us, and we simply allow it. We are not convinced that we deserve better, and we do not have enough confidence in ourselves to go out and find something better, something that we really want. Self-awareness is the key to change. Until we become self-aware, we are oblivious to the fact that the power to change has been and always will be in our own hands – not in the hands of someone else. We can never change until we know who we are today, who we want to be in the future, and when we want to become this new person.

Personal Application:

At the beginning of this chapter, I defined self-awareness as knowing and being able to articulate where you are in your life. I then added that you must also take ownership of and make a commitment to placing yourself on the other side of your situation because you're finally convinced that this is where you belong. Now, I want you to think about the greatest challenge that you overcame, and reflect on the event or series of events that finally convinced you to change your situation. Being as specific as possible, what triggered your enlightenment, and when did this occur? At what point did the pain of remaining the same finally become greater than the pain of changing? How did this happen? What goal(s) were you trying to accomplish? Before proceeding to the next chapter, please take at least 5-10 minutes to answer these questions.

These questions are designed to bring you back to the place where you finally reached the crossroads of decision and indecision. Prior to this point, both your past and your future seemed hopeless. However, due to an unexpected convergence of your positive and negative life experiences that reminded you of the reality that you once knew, while also giving you a renewed confidence in the possibility of experiencing this reality again, you finally arrived at the crossroads of decision and indecision due to this newfound level of self-awareness. Understanding what caused you to become self-aware is essential to understanding the newfound drive, energy, and resourcefulness that followed to help you achieve your goal, especially if you wish to duplicate this process and overcome other life challenges that you may be facing as well. So, consider your trigger, identify what made you want to change, and recall what caused you to remain committed to this process. Do this now.

CHAPTER 6

Healthy Eating: Changing My Philosophy About Food and Changing My Diet

What is food, and what purpose does it serve in my life? Is it my friend, and is it my source of pleasure, comfort and happiness? Or is it my opiate, my addiction, and my escape from reality? Is it the answer to all my problems and my favorite thing to do, or is it my default activity whenever I get bored? Or in reality, is it both my spinach like Popeye and my kryptonite like Superman all at the same time?

At some point in my life, I thought of food in all of these capacities. However, the sad reality is that I have only listed a few. Therefore, as previously stated, to overcome obesity I had to break down my transformation into two steps. The first step dealt directly with the selection and quantity of foods that I had always eaten. Specifically, it spoke to the things that I had to stop doing if I truly desired to lose the weight. I had to STOP eating unhealthy foods and STOP eating in portions that left me feeling swollen and uncomfortable whenever I finished eating. Furthermore, I had to change how I thought about food and what I believed about food as well. Instead of it being a stress reliever for me, I had to understand its true purpose. I had to re-learn that food exists to provide nourishment for the body, and this function is best performed when I eat in moderation, as opposed to gorging myself, at each meal. I had to convince myself that in spite of what I thought, felt, and even what a few of my past experiences may have been, my family was never to going to run out of food, nor was I ever going to go hungry.

At most, I might not be able to get my fill in the manner to which I was accustomed, but never would I go without.

This was huge for me. I learned to accept the reality that less can be more because if I reduced my portion size, my body could actually take in more food over the long run. I also learned to put my situation in perspective because I developed a newfound sensitivity for and awareness of all the people in America and around the world who were homeless and hungry. Somehow, these people were able to survive for an entire week on the same amount of food that I would sometimes eat in one day. So, instead of taking pride in how much food I could eat and how, as I child, I had an appetite that matched or exceeded the appetites of some of the adults in my family, I began to take pride in how little food I could eat before I was full. I began to challenge myself to see how long I could go before I needed to eat again. No longer was I taking pride in family nicknames like "the finisher" or "garbage disposal," nicknames I had earned because I would not only eat my food, but I would also eat whatever anyone else had left over as well. Additionally, instead of taking two or three sandwiches to school each day for both lunch and my after school snack, I eventually began taking pride in the fact that I brought only one sandwich for lunch and ultimately no lunch at all to school. I transitioned from worrying about how hungry I would be by the end of the day, to not worrying about food at all because I knew that I was able to make it through the day just fine.

All of these actions show that when I truly became serious about changing my life and transforming my reality, I had to reconstruct my personal values. In particular, I had to reconstruct my values as it pertains to food. I had to develop the discipline and the determination that would allow my ideas for my future to become my new reality. I also had to learn goal-setting and how to stick to my goals no matter what. Again, this all began the summer after sixth grade. This is when I changed my diet cold turkey by cutting out all foods that were fried, greasy, sweet, carbonated, or otherwise unhealthy, and replaced them with only salads and water for the entire summer. This became my new diet because this was the only way that I thought I could be successful and achieve my goal within my desired timeframe. I was sold out 110% to the idea of becoming skinny, and I was determined to do everything within my power that would help me to achieve this goal. In my mind, there was no time for baby steps or for a gradual process; I needed results *tomorrow* so I could have time to adjust to the new me and be ready for high school. However, I wasn't just preparing myself to attend high school at the small, Christian, private school where I was currently enrolled. I was preparing myself to attend public school – the land flowing with pretty girls and everything else that I wanted. So, drastic times called for drastic measures because I had a point to prove, and this was the most extreme act I could think of. Designing a completely new diet for myself was not as challenging as you may think. Yes, the adjustment was a little rough at first, and yes, I even slipped a few times in the beginning. Nevertheless, I did not let this discourage me nor define who I was. I did not allow my mess-ups to represent the extent of my capabilities. Whenever this would happen, I would assess the situation leading up to my weak moment so I could learn how to not repeat it again; then, I would pick myself up, dust myself off, and try again. It was just like learning how to ride a bicycle for the first time without training wheels. My mental resolve and my laser focus on the objective at hand caused me to persevere and ultimately become successful.

I refer to step one of my two-step transformation as "Healthy Eating Habits" because this title presents me with something that I can easily control by simply choosing to not practice poor eating habits any more. My two-step process is all about recognizing and taking ownership of the things you can control, then working them to your maximum capacity until you can do no more. When you do this, you naturally forget about everything outside of your control, you amplify your focus, and you simplify your process. All these things help you to produce results faster. This is why I found it easier to assume personal responsibility for the foods I that ate, or didn't eat, because this aspect of my life was completely under my control. Making a conscious decision to develop a new diet in place of my old one meant that I had to be positively convinced of the negative effects my old diet was having on my life even though it felt so good every time I ate those foods. So, even though I was not a doctor, nutritionist, or similar health professional, I was a pre-teen who had a very basic understanding that if I ate light foods like salads and water, I would soon become light (skinny) myself. I made this connection because every time I would visit different places or even watch TV, I would always see skinny people eating salads and drinking water. Therefore I made the connection that if it worked for them it will work for me too. So, I cut out everything that I thought had even the slightest chance of making me fat. Changing my diet meant that I had to be totally connected to the fact that the end justified the means, and that no price was too great. It meant that I was willing to find comfort in discomfort because it would all be worth it when I finally arrived. I couldn't wait to be skinny because the majority of my life thus far had been lived as a fat person.

Making these connections and putting my blinders on to block out any and all distractions that might come my way was actually a lot easier than I thought. Before long, my body started reflecting the fact that I had changed the foods that I was putting into it: My stomach didn't stick out as much and my clothing size actually went down. I was especially excited about my clothing size reduction because instead of being limited to only the "husky" section whenever we went shopping, I now had other options. What's more, all of this began to happen within just a few short weeks. Now, I'm not saying that I completely lost all my weight that summer, but I am saying that I made significant progress. In fact, I made so much progress that my confidence skyrocketed, and I became even more committed to achieving my goal. Through discipline and determination I was able to set my goals and stick to them in the face of my family and everyone else around me who still practiced the poor eating habits to which I was previously accustomed. They did not know what I was doing or what my true intentions were, and yet I succeeded.

My process started out as an experimental journey. I began by eating salads only two times a day, but I soon realized that I needed another meal. So, I moved to eating salads three times a day: one for breakfast, one for lunch and one for dinner. At first I would eat lettuce only, but eventually I started being more creative and colorful with my salads by adding whatever I could find in the refrigerator: eggs, fruit, meat, different vegetables, different salad dressings, and the like. There was no right or wrong way to do it because I was making it up as I went along. All I knew was that I was eating my salads, and I was having fun while I was doing it. I was totally in control, and this motivated me even more. This went on for the entire summer. I really appreciated this kick-start that I gave myself because it truly set the stage for my journey. It let me know that all things are possible if I simply set my mind to it – even if it means taking on my current greatest challenge. Since I had always been a good student in the classroom who made straight A's all through elementary school, I was somewhat familiar with the concepts of self-discipline, self-determination and hard work. However, it wasn't until that summer following the sixth grade that I was finally able to expand my understanding of these three concepts beyond the classroom and apply them to a real-life situation. It wasn't until that summer that I was finally ready to take ownership of and pursue mastery over the fact that the same things I did to be successful in the classroom would also be required for me to be successful in other areas of my life as well. In summary, it was this change in my philosophy on life that caused me to change how I think about food, change my diet, and develop the healthy eating habits that I still practice to this day.

Personal Application:

When you finally resolved to change your situation and to overcome your former greatest challenge, what action steps did you take? What plan did you establish for yourself, and how did you execute this plan? What newfound realizations did you make that clarified and simplified the steps you had to take to get from where you were to where you wanted to be? What goal(s) were you trying to accomplish? Describe the first 90 days following your decision in as much detail as you can remember. What were some of your early successes and some of your early failures? How did they affect you? Did you have to change any of your long-held thoughts and beliefs? Did your personal values shift or evolve during this process? In what areas did you learn to find comfort through discomfort because you knew it would all be worth it in the end?

This chapter officially marks the beginning of the second half of the book, and this portion of the book is dedicated to taking action. The content in this half is intentionally written to be more personal in order to facilitate deeper levels of self-reflection. More questions will be asked of you as you continue reading, and these questions will focus specifically on extracting information from you that you probably haven't thought about in a very long time. The intent is to help you illuminate the road that you traveled to find your Sweetest Victory so you can be reminded of how great you truly are, and so you can use this road map again in the future. Therefore, please don't hesitate, skip over, or otherwise procrastinate when it comes to answering any of the questions that are asked of you in this Personal Application or in any of the following chapters either. So, before you proceed, grab your notebook and begin answering these questions now.

CHAPTER 7

Exercise and Fitness: Changing My Lifestyle

Step two in my transformation came when I decided to incorporate physical activity into my life. The moment I realized that I must change my diet if I wanted to lose weight, I also realized that I must begin exercising as well if I wanted to "get ripped" and experience long-lasting results in the shortest amount of time possible. I understood that doing one without the other would be like rowing a boat with just one oar: I'd be exerting a lot of energy only to find myself going in circles and getting nowhere. So, by focusing again only on the things I could control, the things that I knew, and the things that were within my reach, I decided to create a personal exercise regimen to accompany my new eating habits. My goal was to challenge myself to do something I had never done before because I needed results as soon as possible. Therefore, I envisioned the most extreme exercise plan I could think of, and I set this as my goal so I could begin working out according to this plan immediately. These are the goals that I committed to doing each day: perform 500 sit-ups, perform 500 push-ups, run at least 5 laps around the block, and maintain this regimen for at least 5 days a week throughout the entire summer.

Of course when I first started, and even by the end of the summer, I wasn't able to complete 500 sit-ups or 500 push-ups all at one time. So, I began this process incrementally, starting off with sets of 5 to 10 push-ups and 5 to 10 sit-ups at a time because I literally was not able to perform one complete sit-up or one standard push-up when I first began. I had to struggle and fight my way through this process daily by doing things that were not easy, things that did not feel good, things that caused me to lose my breath, and things that caused me to sweat profusely, all by the fifth repetition. My self-proclaimed weight room was my grandmother's hallway, and her Del Paso Heights neighborhood was my jogging circuit. This is where it all went down for me. By the end of the summer, I would eventually get to the point where I could successfully perform 75 sit-ups and 75 push-ups at one time. I made it this far because each and every time that I was able to complete five repetitions with even the slightest sense of ease, I would always push myself to add five more repetitions so I would never get comfortable. Getting comfortable was totally unacceptable for me because I wanted to break myself from thinking that everything in life was supposed to be comfortable; in fact, I conditioned myself to believe that being comfortable was my enemy. I did not want to rest because I felt that each moment I rested, my goal of becoming skinny was slipping farther and farther away from me, and I just had to have it. That's why I always pushed myself to work so hard because I truly believed that becoming thin was only within my reach if I stayed focused and gave it my all each and every day. This was literally the only hope that I had as a twelve-year-old boy.

Imagine this, with each sit-up attempt, you only make it a quarter of the way, or at best halfway up, before gravity kicks in and brings you crashing back down to the ground because your stomach is so big and it's always in your way. Your stomach begins to feel like an immovable barrier that is preventing your elbows from making contact with your knees. Therefore, completing each set of sit-ups feels like nothing more than a mere fantasy to you, almost like reaching for the brass ring that's too far out of reach as you're stuck on a never-ending merry-go-round. Simultaneously, you feel like you could enter cardiac arrest at any moment because with each sit-up attempt you feel as though you are literally crushing your lungs. Shortness of breath ensues, and thoughts like: "I can't do it. It's too hard. This isn't fair. Why do I have to be so fat anyway? I feel like I'm going to die. I don't know if I'm ever going to get skinny. Is there any other way? I'm never going to be able to do this." begin to plague your mind. All of this happened to me in the beginning. I felt as if the task I had set out to accomplish was too much for me to overcome. I felt this way quite regularly because in the same way that I had changed my eating habits cold turkey, I had similarly jumped into the deep end with my workout regimen as well because I had never worked out before in my entire life. Nevertheless, I resolved that I was either going to sink or swim because success was my only option. Even though negative thoughts and the idea of quitting came to mind, it felt as if I had a guardian angel that would immediately spring into action in these moments and tell me that I could do it. It would always remind me of my ultimate goal. It would encourage me to focus on the fact that even though it was hard for me right then, if I just kept trying, it would eventually be possible for me to do a sit-up as long as I didn't give up. These moments represented some of my first and most memorable encounters with my alter ego, which I refer to as the Voice of Reason, and it didn't take long for me to realize that its singular objective was to help me become the person that I was destined to be.

At different points in our lives, I believe that the person we are today will subconsciously encounter the person we are destined to be in the future. If we expect to go to the next level personally, professionally, spiritually, socially, or otherwise, we must focus on developing within ourselves the specific attributes and characteristics of our future selves that we currently do not possess. We must focus on developing the attributes and characteristics that are revealed to us through these subconscious encounters. Whenever we make up our minds to deliberately pursue the person that we are destined to be, the Voice of Reason comes to us at the most opportune moments in our journey when we are at the crossroads of a destiny-shaping decision. It's in these moments, when we have clearly defined our goals and when we have been impassioned to relentlessly pursue them that the Voice of Reason comes to counsel us on the things that we should and should not do. We always have the choice to listen or not to listen, but understand that this counsel only comes to inform us of the things that will either draw us closer to or further away from the whole person that we are destined to be.

For me, the Voice of Reason has assumed several prominent figures in my life as I was pursuing various goals that were extremely important to me. For example, during my transition from fat to fit, I envisioned the Voice of Reason as a coach roaring at me, telling me what I must do to develop self-discipline, and holding me accountable for doing these things daily. During college, I envisioned the Voice of Reason as a spotting partner who was there to help me lift the heavy load of my classes, along with my other responsibilities as well, when things got too hard, when things got too heavy, and when I felt like giving up on completing my degree. Now, as I'm building my business, the Voice of Reason assumes the role of a highly successful executive and inspirational specialist who coaches me and reminds me of things such as: achievement knows no excuses, manage your priorities and your actions so they always remain consistent with achieving your magnificent obsession, and maintain a laser focus that's unwavering and unapologetic in its execution. Let's resume our football story:

> We are now at the summer entering my sophomore year of high school and I have decided to try football one more time. I was no longer an over-weight, out-of-shape child whose legs rubbed together whenever I walk. I was no longer the child whose favorite snacks were cupcakes, Ho-Ho's, and Snickers. I was no longer the child who always had to have second and third portions. I had since matured into an attractive young man with a well-sculpted body. I had spent the past few summers exercising and eating salads to drop the weight because I was determined to improve my physical appearance. Additionally, I was preparing myself for another, more successful encounter with football because this time I was not going to be denied. I still loved football, and my primary motivation was to prove to myself that I was not a quitter. Even

though I might have made a regretful decision in the past, I was not about to let that happen again, nor was I going to let it define who I was or what I could be.

In high school, I played football for two years. Since then, I have not worked harder physically at any other time in my life. Over the course of those two years, barely a day went by where I did not lift a weight or perform intense callisthenic exercises. A typical day of conditioning would begin in the weight room with strength-training almost to the point of burnout. Then, we would hit the field for cardio. Once we reached the field, it was all over because each day our workout was left up to the coach's discretion. Sometimes we would do stadium runs where everyone on the team would have to run all the stairs in our football stadium multiple times simply because this was "our house." Following stadium runs, we would either do a five-mile run throughout the neighborhood surrounding our high school, hill sprints on the hills surrounding our stadium, suicides up and down the length of the field, or any other creation that our coach would devise for us. We had to do all of this each morning before we would be able to suit up and put on our pads.

Now, picture this: 100+ degree weather, helmets, shoulder pads, thigh pads and cleats. Then, add sit-ups, leg lifts, bicycle kicks, up-downs, push-ups, scissor runs, wind sprints, tackling drills, and the list goes on and on. Some combination of all these things occurred almost daily as a part of our conditioning process before we would ever line up in formation and begin running plays. My coach's favorite sayings were: "You are going to be the most well-conditioned team on the field," and that "You should be in good enough shape to play four more quarters of football even after the first four quarters were over." In particular, he also drove home the importance of still being able to give 100% in the fourth quarter, even after three quarters of football, because this is when everyone else usually gets tired. He believed that it was in the fourth quarter where the game was won, and he tried his best to get us to understand that.

Of course at that time, most of us did not get it. Instead we all thought our coach was a cross between a half-crazy drill sergeant and a ruthless dictator who loved to yell senseless rhetoric at us. At that time, most of us were struggling just to make it through all the drills, and I know I was for sure. Yes, there were times when I wanted to give up. There were times when I was so out of breath I had to lean all the way over to the ground so that I could pull oxygen from the grass because my lungs weren't doing the trick by themselves. There were even times when I threw up from running so hard. With everything that I was going through, I could have easily given up and allowed this football experience to turn out the same way my previous experience did, but this time my mind was made up. Even though I was not a Christian at the time, the spirit of the Biblical admonition to "run with patient endurance and steady persistence the appointed course of the race that is set before [me]" was very much my driving force. Quitting was not an option for me. Therefore, I was resolved and determined to give all that I had in this fight of my life. I was *literally* going to run this race in order to keep myself from being sidelined again because I had to make it to Friday night under the lights.

This is what made all the suffering worthwhile for me, especially as a varsity football player. The rush, the energy, the crowd, the exhilarating sense of liberty that came over me when our team marched on the track surrounding the field in our teal and black uniforms, when we sprinted onto the field through the welcome tunnel of junior varsity football players and cheer leaders that had

> been made for us underneath the scoreboard, and when we did our infamous "Husky Jacks" jumping jacks on the 50-yard line with the entire stadium in an uproar rooting us on and our award-winning marching band playing their ever-famous "fight music" in the background. This was all worth it for me. Many of us knew that high school would be the extent of our football careers, so each Friday night home game was like our own mini Super Bowl, or at least was for me.

More than 14 years removed from when I first began my transition from fat to fit, I now have tremendous difficulty remembering many of the dominant thoughts that literally brought me to the verge of giving up because the process was getting too hard. In the beginning, I did think about giving up quite often. However, after giving myself over to the guidance of my alter ego and submitting completely to the Voice of Reason, the majority of my memories were always like this: "No matter how hard it may get, I'm not going to quit. I'm going to prove to myself that I'm not a quitter. I'm going to be a star athlete on the football team if I just keep trying. The girls are going to love me, love my body, and they won't be able to keep their hands off of me." Since thoughts like these dominated my mind, I refused to allow any other thoughts outside of my school work to enter in because I didn't have the capacity to entertain anything else. This first began as a series of conscious decisions that I made regularly. However, before I knew it this process was happening automatically. It was as if my mind and my will had come into alignment, and they were subconsciously safeguarding themselves against all thoughts that weren't consistent with my ultimate goal. As a result, I began to notice several changes that were taking place in my life. One major change was that I had greatly enhanced my peer group selection. I had begun hanging out with people who enjoyed doing things that did not revolve around eating, and by the time I got to high school, I had begun spending more time with my fellow football players and other friends who valued working out as much as I did. Working out was becoming an all-consuming passion for me, and I did not have time nor did I have the desire to hang with people who did not share my same values. My priorities were: working out, hanging out with the ladies, and my school work because this was always important to me despite all the other changes that were happening in my life. As I drew closer and closer to the fulfillment of my ultimate desire, my lifestyle naturally adapted because I had given myself over to the Voice of Reason so it could guide me towards becoming the healthy person that I was destined to be.

Personal Application:

Have you ever had a Voice of Reason experience? Have you ever encountered a time in your life where an unexplainable yet powerful internal compass guided you and counseled you on the way that you should go during a moment of complete uncertainty? Think back and recall these moments. As you reflect, I also want you to recall an area of your life that you were extremely motivated to improve and further develop at one particular point in time. This can be anything from your health, to your education, to your personal relationships, or any other area of your life. All that's important is that you were successful in either achieving or exceeding your self-improvement goal(s) for whatever area you choose. I want you to focus on this area like a laser. In the moments, days, weeks, months, or even years leading up to you accomplishing your goal, whenever it seemed too tough and you felt like giving up, what were some of the unexpected safeguards that were triggered in your mind to keep you focused and on task? What safeguards were triggered when it seemed like things were not going to work out for you? What did you hear and what were you reminded of in these moments?

Now, let's use some of these same questions to better understand how you overcame your greatest challenge. When you first started out, how did you develop your solution for accomplishing your goal? What specific life adjustments occurred automatically as you were pursuing your goal? Once you finally gained enough courage to face what you were afraid of, what enabled you to stay in the fight and ultimately achieve success? When it got hard along the way, what motivated you to keep going and not give up? Did anyone tell you to do this? Did anyone else know about your situation and what you were doing to change it? Did you have an external support system to assist you and encourage you along the way?

Before you advance to the final chapter, please take some time and give thoughtful consideration to each of the questions presented here. By now, you should have clearly identified the greatest challenge of your past, gained new insights on the magnitude of this feat, and been reminded of how amazing you truly are. When you bring all of this together, there are only two questions that yet remain: "Does my life today still reflect the greatest challenge that I overcame in my past?" and "What lessons can I learn from my past that are also applicable to any other challenge that I am currently facing?" Let's proceed.

CHAPTER 8

Healthy Living: Maintaining and Moving Forward

Doing something once can be considered an accident. Doing something twice can be considered lucky. However, doing something three or more times consecutively can represent a definitive and strategic skill set that is superior in nature to other people who are aspiring for the same goal. Or, it can also mean that you're crazy! For the purposes of this discussion though, let's assume it's the former and not the latter. Does my life today still reflect the fact that I overcame childhood obesity, and do I live in such a way that I honor the legacy of what I have accomplished? Are my eating habits, exercise habits, and attitudes about food still the same today as they were when I first made my transition? Have I shown youth who struggle with childhood obesity how to overcome this challenge? Have I shown others how to overcome their greatest challenge even if they struggled with something else other than their weight? How have I taken what I've learned and applied it to other areas of my life, and what additional lessons did overcoming obesity teach me?

As I think about my final words of inspiration that I want to leave with you as both a call to action and a source of personal reflection, all these questions come to mind. More than 10 years removed from my peak physical condition and more than 14 years removed from my initial transition from fat to fit, this book has just now been written. First physically, then socially and emotionally, it took me a long time to overcome childhood obesity and all the direct and indirect consequences that it had on my life. I hope this book has given you an inside look into the life of an obese youth and allowed you to understand many of the challenges that obese youth everywhere deal with each day: the bad, the ugly, and the unthinkable. Similarly, I hope this book has been an encouragement for you as you learned about the process that I went through to overcome childhood obesity and eliminate all traces of this psychological disorder from my life. I am proud to say that my life today does not indicate that I ever battled with obesity during my childhood, and you would never know this about me unless I told you or unless you knew me when I was a child. For this I am extremely grateful to God because to this day, whenever I tell people that I battled with childhood obesity, they rarely believe me unless I show them pictures of how I used to look as proof. My eating and exercise habits are not as extreme as they used to be, but they are still very much controlled. Currently, I work out at least 3 days a week, and if I'm not able to make it to the gym I work out at home. Moreover, my attitude towards food is still very much the same. I yet eat several small meals in moderation throughout the day, and I still refrain from eating many of the unhealthy foods that I mentioned in Chapter 6. All of this is important because collectively, it was all of these things that led me to discovering the two greatest lessons my process of overcoming childhood obesity has taught me. First, I learned that our circumstances are the key to us becoming the person we are destined to be. And second, I learned that my purpose in life is to harness and unleash the power of my life story so I can help others overcome something that I already overcame. At the core of my entire experience from pre-obese, to obese, to post-obese, these two lessons ring true for me in very resounding ways because I have been able to connect so many things to these two foundational ideas. As I share these truths, I will further expound upon my life lessons, and I will provide in-depth responses to the questions I posed in the beginning of the chapter.

Lesson 1: Our circumstances are the key to us becoming the person we are destined to be. There are times in our life when we find ourselves in seemingly unexplainable and virtually unbeatable situations that have our backs completely against the wall, and there's no way out or no way to escape anywhere in sight. In these moments, many people give up, retreat, or otherwise back down from the situation in surrender and in acknowledgement that the situation is too great. Whenever this happens, "surrendering" usually means one of two things: It's a short-term solution that's applied in order to regroup and gather the proper reinforcements to get back into the fight as soon as possible. Or, it's a long-term, almost permanent reality that's willingly accepted, similar to how I wallowed in the depths of despair during my obesity years because I didn't believe that I could change my situation.

For six long years I lived as a victim of my environment, but here's an even more shocking thought that could have easily become my reality: if my circumstances had been any lighter or even slightly more bearable, I could have easily remained an obese youth for another six years or more. Nevertheless, because I didn't see my situation easing up anytime soon, in the summer following the sixth grade I decided that I had enough and that now was the best time to begin transforming my life. Often misunderstood and rarely ever appreciated, our life circumstances are almost always tailor-made just for us. They are designed to provoke us in ways that will get us to move and keep us supplied with the energy and the inspiration that we need to not grow weary during our time of transformation. It's not until our circumstances have penetrated our very core and are actively disrupting our inner peace with no apparent end or lessening of the pain in sight that we finally become ready and willing to commit ourselves to taking consistent action. When we finally commit ourselves at this level, our commitment to action will typically continue for as long as it takes to permanently change our situation. The pain had finally become unbearable for me, and I was not going to allow my future to be doomed before it had a chance to be written.

Achieving your potential requires major personal sacrifices in many different areas of your life in order to successfully become the person that you are destined to be. This process is not easy, nor is it supposed to be. This time of refining means undoing the many years of bad habits and poor practices that you've developed over your lifetime, and replacing them with new habits and improved practices that will make you a better person. Without a crystal-clear understanding of what you're leaving behind and why you're leaving it, your motivation to accomplish your new goal will be wavering at best. In addition, you will be left wondering why your ultimate goal is always evading you. At this point, I can honestly say that I am grateful that I battled with childhood obesity. Childhood obesity was entrusted to me, and I count it a privilege and an honor to have been worthy enough to bear this challenge. For me, this meant that something even greater was placed inside of me that would eventually help me to overcome it. Furthermore, I would also be able to show others how to overcome obesity and ultimately show people everywhere how to harness and unleash the power of their life stories as well so they too could duplicate this process in other areas of their lives. Therefore, it is for these reasons that I say that our circumstances are the key to us becoming the person we are destined to be and why I believe that we all should be thankful for all the circumstances that we've encountered in our lives.

Lesson 2: My purpose in life is to harness and unleash the power of my life story so I can help others overcome something that I already overcame. Writing this book required that I travel down a path of self-discovery that I had never traveled down before. It required that I be willing to engage some of the most sensitive areas of my life in order to induce my healing and enable me to share with others some of the most important lessons that I learned along the way. This process challenged me to engage areas of my life that I initially wanted to remain hidden forever because I didn't want anyone to know about the parts of my life that caused me to feel extreme shame and disgust. Nevertheless, I consciously decided to fully disclose my "secrets" and allow other people into my intimate zone. I decided to face my fears and re-live some of the most painful experiences in my life just to make sense of my own story so I could understand why these things happened to me, and so I could learn what my experiences were trying to teach me.

Even though this story first began over 20 years ago, I was able to remember each and every step of my journey as if it happened yesterday. I was able to place myself back into those situations socially and emotionally, as both an observer and a participant, and I was able to fully re-acquaint myself with each and every moment and each and every emotion. Even though I cried a lot along the way, I am very proud of my decision to undertake this project because I took so much away from it. How often in our lives do we deliberately enter those old, abandoned, run-down, and dilapidated places in our minds and in our hearts that are boarded up and have been marked "Do Not Enter"? What are we really afraid of? What are we trying to avoid? What are we trying so hard to cover up in the hope that we would someday forget all the unpleasant things that happened to us? Why? Are we afraid that whatever our greatest challenge used to be yet defines aspects of who we are today, and are we embarrassed and ashamed to admit it? Do we believe that people will look at us and treat us differently? Does the pain still run so deep that to even think about this situation is just like pouring salt into an open wound that has never healed? Do you feel that you will lose the very things that you have worked so hard for, and you don't want to chance messing anything up or blowing it? Are you living in such a deep, dark place of denial that you are having trouble even admitting that this situation was ever a part of your life?

Well, this is exactly where I was before writing this book, and this is exactly how I felt about my battle with childhood obesity. I felt this way because I didn't realize that even as an adult, some eight or nine years after being in the peak physical condition of my life and having no physical evidence of ever being an obese youth, I was *still* dealing with the aftermath of childhood obesity and all the social and emotional trauma that it caused me. I can vividly remember the times where I would go off on a rampage and begin ripping up, shredding, and utterly destroying all pictures of myself from my childhood because I couldn't stand to see myself as a fat child. Whenever I would see any school photo, family portrait, or the like, something would come over me and incite this uncontrollable rage within me towards the person that I saw in that picture because that's not who I was any more. That picture did not represent me, I did not want to be mistaken for that person, and I did not want to answer any questions about that time in my life. I tried so desperately to disassociate myself from that person, put as much distance between us as I could, and ultimately eradicate all evidence that this person ever existed. I only wanted people to know me for who I am today, not who I used to be or what I overcame. I carried this stigma with me for many years. I thought that if I looked at those pictures for too long, there was a strong possibility that I might become fat again, and I wasn't going to let that happen. I felt that if people found out about my deep, dark secret, all the girls who had finally started liking me and now wanted to spend time with me, and the measure of coolness and popularity that I had finally gained would all be savagely taken away from me in an instant. I also believed that all the name-calling, ridiculing and fighting that defined my childhood would immediately begin again, and I could not leave this possibility to chance. I had to take decisive actions to ensure that none of this would ever happen again. However, I took these actions at the expense of being yelled at and getting in trouble by my mom because I was destroying all of "her" pictures.

To me, destroying these pictures was worth the risk of getting in trouble because my logic was I could deal with my mom being mad at me, but I couldn't deal with losing the new image that I had worked so hard to create for myself because this would be something from which I could never recover. All hope would be lost for me, and this would probably be the case for the rest of my life. Fortunately though, these destructive tantrums only occurred during high school, and I have since matured. However, here I am as an adult finally having to face and conquer all of these deep-seated fears that I have maintained since my early childhood just so I could move on from one chapter to the next as I wrote this book. So, to say that this task was tough for me is an understatement, but I knew I had no other choice.

The idea of harnessing and unleashing the power of my life story didn't hit me until somewhere around Chapter 2. Prior to this point, I had decided to write my life story simply because I had begun using parts of it as the subject of my morning assembly talks at the high school where I was teaching. Naturally, I elected to share my own story with the students, as opposed to some other topic, because it helped me to better relate with them. It also gave me instant credibility whenever I talked to them about controversial topics because they knew I had been through something in my life just like they had. However, while writing Chapter 2, I realized that both locally and nationally, the childhood obesity epidemic had really started receiving a lot of attention. There were so many notable people like First Lady Michelle Obama and notable organizations like The California Endowment that were directing a lot of resources towards addressing this issue. Observing this trend and the fact that so many different stories about this epidemic had started surfacing as well, I immediately began to feel special and important. I had overcome the very thing that all these people and all these entities were trying so diligently to help other people overcome. A renewed sense of purpose and inspiration had come over me almost instantly. Furthermore, I also received the following revelation: Since I had overcome childhood obesity, this meant that I could now show other obese youth how to do the same thing as well. I could harness and unleash the power of my life story for this specific audience because I was uniquely qualified to do so. As a result, I was compelled to take action because I wanted to show how much more effective obesity intervention could be if the people and the entities with resources were more deliberate about equipping the people and the entities who had first-hand experience with everything they needed to do the work.

So, I reached out to one of my mentors, Chet P. Hewitt, President of the Sierra Health Foundation in Sacramento, CA, for support. He gave me a mini-grant to pilot my obesity intervention program at a local middle school where I would be able to implement my program for overweight and obese youth in order to help them develop healthier lifestyles. The objectives of the program were simple: to help urban youth understand that childhood obesity is a psychological disorder with physical consequences, and to equip them with the tools they needed to overcome their greatest challenge. The program focused on strengthening self-esteem, instilling self-determination, and empowering students to no longer remain victims of their circumstances. In addition, through our partnership with the Sacramento Association of Black Social Workers (SABSW), the program engaged parents as well because we wanted to educate all guardians and providers on how to best support and encourage their children during this time of transition. All of this was achieved through the use of Motivational Intervention (M.Int.), and as a result, the program was an amazing success. The name of the program was "The Sweetest Victory," and the school that I chose was Will C. Wood Middle School in Sacramento, CA. Both school officials and officials from the district office loved the program. By the time we finished, we had received several inquiries and requests to expand the program on an even larger level to other middle schools and high schools within the Sacramento City Unified School District. So, here are a few highlights from our 60-Day program:

- The students increased their beliefs in the amount of control they had over their lives by 23%, their knowledge of weight management techniques by 25%, and the frequency with which they practice Healthy Habits by 52%.
- The students gave an average satisfaction rating of 87.38% for each program session, and their favorite parts of the program were: the inspirational speeches, the personal interviews, and the food.
- The greatest sustained weight loss experienced by a single student was 6lbs.
- During the program, the students reported an average of 23 days where they ate at least 5 servings of fruits and vegetables.

- The students logged a total of 2,740 minutes of daily physical activity over and above the time they spent in PE each day during the 60 days of the program.

As evidenced by the "The Sweetest Victory," harnessing and unleashing the power of my life story is more than just a good idea to me. I refer to this process as my purpose in life because I am passionate about doing this work, I believe that I can be the best in the world at doing this work, and doing this work provides me with an extreme sense of fulfillment. Sharing the story of how I overcame childhood obesity and illuminating each step that I took along the way energizes people to do the exact same thing. When I present myself as an example of someone who has transitioned from fat to fit, I stand before them as proof positive that they too can overcome their greatest challenge and transform it into their Sweetest Victory – which for me, was overcoming childhood obesity.

Even though my story is specific to childhood obesity, many of my speaking engagements today have me in front of young professionals, corporations, associations, and even overweight and obese adults because I present my story in a way that's relevant and meaningful to each audience. Harnessing and unleashing the power of your life story is something that's universal, and I would love to see each and every person do this in all aspects of their lives: personal, professional, civic, social, and the like. When people achieve mastery of this process, they will find themselves able to accomplish many tasks, great and small, that they previously may have struggled to overcome. Furthermore, they will overcome these challenges with fluidity and ease. The benefits of learning to harness and unleash the power of your life story include: increased efficiency, productivity, and profitability; increased earning potential; enhanced opportunities for upward mobility; enhanced interpersonal relations; stronger critical thinking skills; greater self-confidence; amplified focus and personal discipline; sustained weight loss; a renewed commitment to consistent and deliberate action; and a greater level of fulfillment, morale and engagement in the work that you do, just to name a few.

As I close, I'm going to leave you with a few practical ideas that I've found to be true based on my own life experiences. I challenge you to apply these ideas towards your own life as well if you desire to go to the next level and if you desire to become the person that you are destined to be. These are the principles that I live by, and I still find them to be just as effective for me today as they were when I first discovered them over 12 years ago:

1. **Create a clear mental picture of what success looks like for you, and envision yourself achieving this goal at least 10 times a day** - At all times, I maintained an extremely detailed mental picture of how I wanted my body to look based on pictures from men's health magazines and fitness commercials that I saw on TV. This mental picture became an all-consuming passion for me to the point where it was all that I thought about. Furthermore, I made sure that all my actions were consistent with drawing me closer towards achieving this goal. This intense level of belief and absolute clarity is what made the pain of changing not only bearable but worth it for me because I knew that where I wanted to be was so much greater than where I currently was. This mental picture, along with visions of women flocking to me because I was "cute, sexy, hot, etc..." is what kept me motivated.

2. **Decide. Believe. Take Action. Repeat.** – It all began with a decision. First and foremost, I made up my mind that I was no longer going to be fat anymore after more than six long years of being obese and enduring all the painful experiences that came along with it. Then, I began believing that it was possible for me to be skinny and that I could once again enjoy fun and desirable interactions with women. From there, I took action on the things I could control: I cut out all the unhealthy foods that I previously loved to eat, replaced them with healthier food choices, and I placed myself on a strict exercise regimen where I committed to do a certain amount of physical activity each

day. So, if you believe something long enough, visualize it clearly enough, and work at it hard enough, it will come to pass.

3. **<u>Unlock your power and activate your magnificent obsession</u>** – All too often we live life unaware of the tremendous amount of personal power that we possesses when we finally decide to make up our minds and do something. This power is unleashed only when we develop an unwavering and unapologetic commitment to accomplishing something that's very specific. The power of a personal belief, emotionalized to the point that it becomes a deep-seated, personal conviction has the power to sustain us and keep us on course even when everything else is telling us that we should stop trying and just give up. In order for a life-transforming change to occur, we must give ourselves over to this process fully and completely. Nothing less will do. Anything less will not generate enough momentum for us to build and maintain continual progress. Therefore, we're wasting our time if we're not willing to give our all to the process because this process must become our magnificent obsession. Becoming skinny was my personal conviction, and having positive interactions with girls was my magnificent obsession.

4. **<u>Challenge the odds and invest in the unproven</u>** – Even though I've accomplished many important things since then, the time in my life when I felt most successful was when I overcame childhood obesity. Beating obesity represented something that I had never done before, and there was no external evidence suggesting that I would ever be successful at it outside of my own personal belief and desire. So, when I reflect on the amount of time, energy, and effort that was required for me to lose the weight and obtain a body that I was proud of, overcoming my unhealthy lifestyle and freeing myself from my unhealthy way of thinking is clearly one of the most powerful

decisions of my entire life. I invested in myself even though what I was planning to do was unproven. I developed a new form of obesity intervention, and used it to escape the undiagnosed grips of two well-known psychological disorders, Binge Eating Disorder and Body Dysmorphic Disorder. I beat the odds, and I yielded the return of a lifetime!

5. **Find a support group** - In the beginning, I did everything alone. However, as time went on I was fortunate enough to be a part of some very intense PE classes, and from there I started playing football. From these group-oriented activities, I learned many valuable lessons about the benefits of working in a team of like-minded individuals, and I want to share my top three:

    - You will constantly be challenged to perform better
    - You will be reminded to stay focused
    - You will be held accountable for your results

    I call this the "winning environment" because you will immediately notice yourself experiencing greater levels of success when you join a support group that is just as committed to you achieving your goals as you are.

6. **For the fastest results, become resolved sooner** - The single greatest factor that could have sped up my process was for me to have made up my mind sooner that I was no longer going to be fat and that I was no longer going to accept a reality that I did not want for myself. Even though it took me almost three years to finally get the body that I wanted, I endured the pain of being an obese youth for more than six years prior to this point simply because I allowed it to happen. I felt powerless over my situation. I didn't know how to change it, and I didn't believe that change was possible. This nine-year transformation could have easily been reduced down to seven years, six years,

five years, four years or maybe even less if I had simply become resolved sooner.

After all of this, here is my final question: What's your story, and are you using it productively in your own life? In reading this book, I not only hope that you've connected with my story, but I also hope this book has prompted you to give serious thought and consideration to your own story as well. The principles discussed in this book can easily be applied across many different disciplines, professions, and situations. They can also serve as an outline to help you re-create your own roadmap to success, one that you have already proven to be effective in your own life. My ultimate desire is that you challenge yourself to pursue mastery at overcoming your greatest challenge and transforming it into your Sweetest Victory on a consistent basis. When you become proficient at this and you are able to do this repeatedly, you will have unconsciously built your own monument of success and fulfillment that no one can ever take from you because you would have finally uncovered the roadmap to *your* Sweetest Victory.

ABOUT THE AUTHOR

For the last eight years, Amos Nugent III has been inspiring people all across this country from the San Francisco Bay Area to Washington, DC. In an effort to help people maximize their potential and uncover the significance of their life story, he has spoken to thousands about the connection that exists between these two ideas and how they directly influence your level of personal success. Amos presents his case to youth and adults on Overcoming Obesity, Overcoming Your Greatest Challenge, and Success Strategies for School, Life and Work as his topics of choice because they best leverage his personal experience. As a professional communicator, Amos Nugent III takes great pride in using this most captivating art form to provide multi-sensory experiences that connect with people in relevant and engaging ways. Amos helps people understand that all they need to do to move from where they are now to where they want to be is simply look within.

As someone who battled childhood obesity for many years but successfully overcame this monumental life struggle by simply resolving that he was no longer going to accept this reality for his life, Amos has spoken before many audiences about Managing Emotions and Thriving Under Pressure, Goal-Setting and Time Management, and Discomfort or Destiny: Can I See the Best in Me? He has been asked to keynote graduation ceremonies, leadership retreats, educational summits, and other similar events. In addition, Amos is also a national speaker with Monster's Making It Count, and he has spoken to thousands of high school students all across the country. Most notably, as a graduate of Howard University, Amos has been invited to speak at the campus of his alma mater several times for many different occasions including prayer breakfasts, freshman orientations, and awards ceremonies.

Additionally, as a native of Sacramento, CA, Amos Nugent III has been recognized for his work in his home community as an advocate for higher education, a professional communicator, and as an entrepreneur by the Observer Media Group as one of the Sacramento Region's "30 Under 30" most promising young leaders. He is also a Senior Fellow of the Nehemiah Emerging Leaders Program (NELP), and he proudly serves on the board of directors for the United College Action Network (UCAN) and the Women's Civic Improvement Club (WCIC).

Currently, Amos Nugent III serves as a Vice Principal for Community Collaborative Charter School (Robertson Center), the Founder and Managing Director of Spoken Life LLC, and he is also the President of Enlightened Minds Group Inc. Amos Nugent III regularly shares his story through keynotes and workshops at seminars, conferences, school assemblies and other live events. If this information has piqued your interest, feel free to contact Amos directly to find out how you can experience him in person!

For more information on booking Amos to come and speak at your next event or to bring the "The Sweetest Victory" to your group, please visit: www.amosnugent.com.

Made in the USA
Monee, IL
04 November 2026

67381732R00049